Efficacy of Velvet Antler in Veterinary Practice

PJ Broadfoot, D.V.M.

Nina Anderson, S.P.N.

Safe Goods Publishing

Authors:

PJ Broadfoot, D.V.M.

Attended Kansas State University, Manhattan, KS and obtained a BS in Animal Science and Industry, with an emphasis on Genetics. Graduated KSU School of Veterinary Medicine 1981, Cum Laude. She started a solo practice in Van Buren, AR in 1982. PJ is married to Jeff Broadfoot, and has four grown children, Brannon, Barrett, Burke and Brea. Member of the Arkansas Veterinary Medical Association, American Veterinary Medical Association, American Holistic Veterinary Medicine. She is a Board Member of the American Society of Bioregulatory Medicine (ASBRM) Registration of Alternative and Integrative Veterinary Education (RAIVE) board member Instructor College of Integrative Veterinary Technologies (CIVT) an international online college. She has given lectures on nutritional aspects of healing, and the influence of environment and nutrition on children with learning and behavior difficulties. PJ lectures extensively on Complimentary Medicine in U.S and abroad. Published articles have been included in such diverse journals as Explore Magazine, The AHVMA Journal, The Biotherapy Journal, distributed in the U.S. and Germany, and The Integrative Veterinary Care Journal. She co-authored a textbook: *Integrating Complementary Medicine into Veterinary Practice* (Wiley Blackwell 2008)

Nina Anderson, S.P.N., C.NLP, C.NLH

Nina is a Specialist in Performance Nutrition, a certified Neurolinguistic Programmer and Reiki practitioner. She has been an active researcher in the alternative health field for over twenty years and has co-authored 18 books on holistic health including *Are You Poisoning Your Pets, The Electric Pet* and *Super Nutrition for Dogs n' Cats.* She is President of LJB Piper, a company that makes an electrolyte concentrate supplement. She has appeared on numerous national radio and TV shows and has been a feature columnist for several holistic trade magazines.

ISBN 9781634527590
Library of Congress Catalog in Publication: 2015936266
Printed in the United States of America

Published by Safe Goods
561 Shunpike Rd.
Sheffield, MA 01257
888 217-7233

Efficacy of Velvet Antler in Veterinary Practice **is** not intended as medical advice. No claims are made for the ability of products mentioned to treat, cure or prevent any disease. No promise is made for health, and no diagnostic or health claims are stated. This literature is for informational purposes only and is not meant to diagnose, or prescribe for any health condition. Always see a veterinarian for matters relating to your pet's health. The FDA has not evaluated this information.

Table of Contents

Chapter One — 7
Snapshot of the efficacy of Deer Velvet Antler in Animals.

Chapter Two — 13
The Many Uses of Velvet Antler in Veterinary Practice.

Chapter Three — 31
Pharmacology of Velvet Antler

Chapter Four — 35
Velvet Antler for Osteoarthritis – A potential alternative to drugs or surgery

Chapter Five — 41
Clinical Trials and Research

Chapter Six — 53
Velvet Antler – A Word about Cancer

Chapter Seven — 61
Velvet Antler. On the Cutting Edge – Stem Cell Research

Conclusion — 63

Research Directory — 64

Introduction

My commitment to the value of holistic veterinary care for over thirty years, has led me to research the benefit of natural therapies as a beneficial alternative to drug therapy for many clinical conditions that I see in everyday practice. In the past few years, I have discovered that deer velvet is valuable for treating a myriad of illnesses. This remarkable product, particularly when combined with apparent synergists, such as green lipped mussel, thymus, colostrum and others, has helped animals to balance their immune system, recover from joint problems, restore normal skin function, enhance red blood cell production, and improve reproductive activity. Research suggests that it can also benefit those suffering from cardiovascular disease and those recuperating from surgery. We are in serious consideration of how we can incorporate these therapies into a wellness protocol. Think of what we could do, if we improved regenerative capacity and decreased inflammatory conditions in our patients, while they were young! I hope this book can help you understand how important velvet antler can be to the health of your patients and that you will incorporate it as part of your holistic modalities. -PJ Broadfoot DVM

Chapter One

Snapshot of the Efficacy of Deer Velvet Antler in Animals.

Owners of mature cats and dogs are increasingly looking beyond conventional treatments for chronic conditions in their pets, and they appreciate the opportunity for their veterinarian to offer them a broader range of options. They are also looking at wellness treatments to prevent illness and increase vitality. Velvet antler fits well into this range. As a natural therapy backed by robust research, this choice will appeal to many pet owners. Although relatively new to the North American supplement market, velvet antler has been used for centuries by the Asian and Indigenous peoples as a powerful health tonic. This traditional Chinese medicine is a nutritional supplement made from the inner core of deer antler in the velvet stage of growth. Humanely-harvested velvet antler is rapidly becoming a beneficial addition to veterinary healing modalities, including remarkable results in mitigating skin conditions like alopecia.

Common uses for velvet antler encourage:

- Joint function, mobility and arthritis relief
- Alopecia control
- Muscle and connective tissue development and strength
- Immuno-modulation
- Brain development
- Vitality and general wellbeing
- Endurance and durability
- Red blood cell production
- Oxygen carrying capacity
- Speedy tissue recovery/ improved wound healing
- Recuperation after surgery
- Optimal reproductive activity
- Reducing inflammation after injury or exercise
- Cardiovascular health and Diabetes management

The complex proteins and lipids found in velvet antler are thought to provide these health benefits, and continued research is confirming this. Although the main body of research and experience of velvet antler usage applies to humans going back over 2000 years, it is fitting that this knowledge is now being applied to the small animal kingdom by forward thinking vets. In the wild, and prior to domestication, these carnivorous animals relied on the fresh meat, bone and blood of their prey for their health, nutrition and wellness. There is anecdotal evidence that puppies and kittens benefit from velvet antler supplements early in life for skeletal development and strength which helps to prevent the onset of arthritis later in life.

Velvet antler has been used in non-surgical repair of fractures. Examples have been submitted from the Medico-Vet clinic in Israel. Jayden was a nine month old, 36 kg mixed breed dog. Jayden came to the pet medical center after being in a municipal shelter where he was suffering from pain in his hind limb. He was non weight bearing on both hind legs. Radiographs revealed a Trans Acetabular fracture. Jayden received 100 mg Rimadyl and 1500 mg Bioactive Deer Velvet for four weeks. Full recovery was obtained after three weeks.

Before

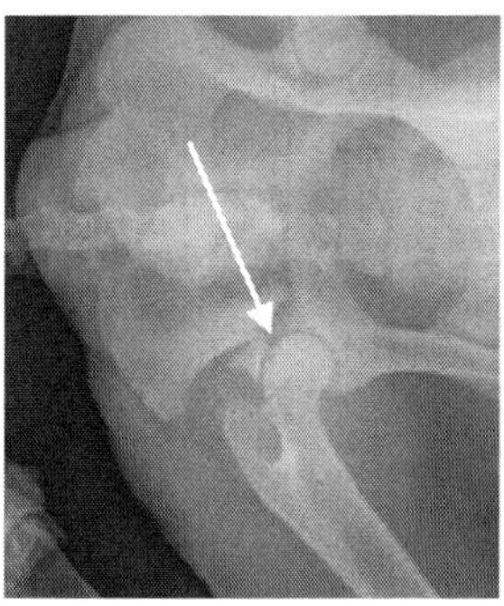

After

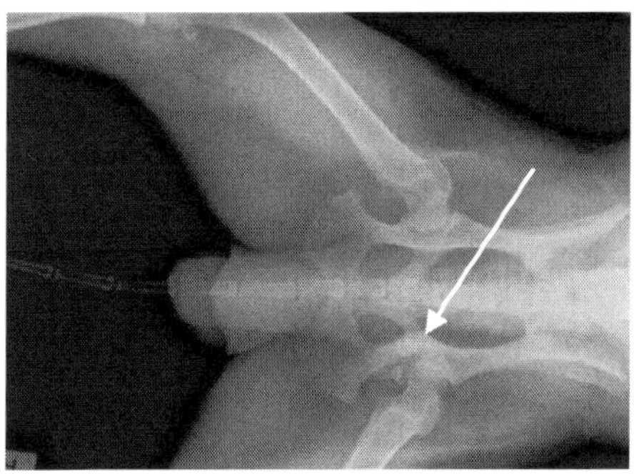

Jack was a one-year-old Pinscher who was brought to the pet medical center with acute trauma to the forelimb. On radiograph, a distal radius and ulna fracture were observed. Non-surgical fixation was done, along with 750 mg Bioactive Deer Velvet. Follow up radiographs after seven days demonstrated an early callus at the fracture site.

Before

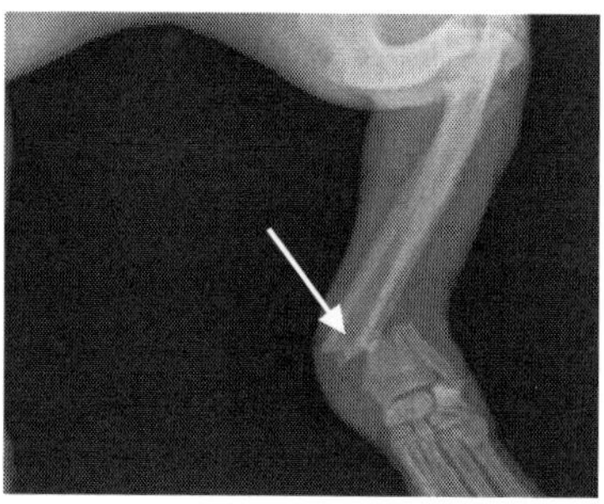

After

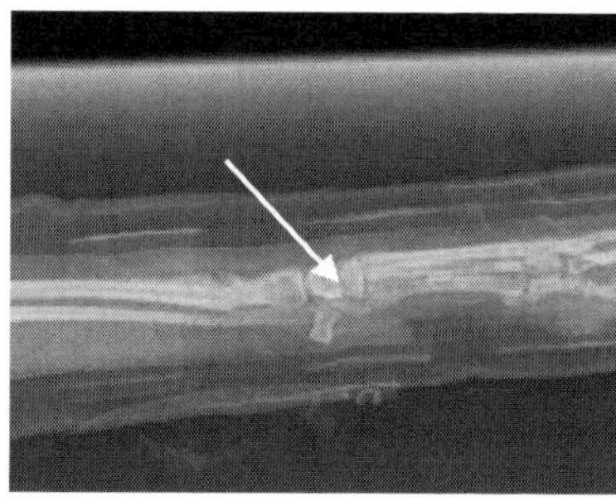

"We've been testing velvet antler on more than 100 small animals with chronic arthritic problems, and the results have been impressive. In more than 80 percent of the cases, we've seen significant improvements in the animal's mobility and vitality.

"We've had dogs come into the hospital that could hardly walk. They were in real pain. But after a couple of

weeks on velvet antler, they're wagging their tail and jumping around. I don't know how often I've heard owners say their pet is acting like a puppy again.

"Unlike human test subjects, who can be influenced by psychological factors, you can't convince an animal that he feels better. He either does or he doesn't. With velvet antler we've seen dramatic improvements that can't be dismissed. And velvet antler doesn't create the kinds of problems we often see with traditional heavy-hitter arthritis drugs that can cause liver damage, kidney damage, bleeding ulcers and a host of other problems.

"As a practicing veterinarian, I'm always a little skeptical of overly-optimistic claims and non-traditional remedies, but velvet antler is the real thing. It's at the top of my list when it comes to treating pets with arthritis and joint pain." — Dr. Clinton Balok, Licensed Veterinarian, Cedar Animal Medical Center, Gallup, N.M. [1]

Cedar Animal Medical Center Clinical Record

Breed	Age	Symp-toms/ Condition	Dosage / Day	Results/Owner Comments
Terrier mix	16	Appetite, activity	200 mg	Improved for 4 months
German Shep-herd	8	Hip pain	200 mg	Improved
Mix	9	Elbows	200 mg	No change in 2 weeks, improvement with 400 mg
Dachshund	12	Hip/back	200 mg	No change
Blue Heeler	7	Neck, back, elbows	210 mg	Improved
Golden Re-triever	11	Appetite, skin, low activity	200 mg	"Great" "new dog"
Lab	10	Hips	200 mg	Improved
Lab	12	Hips, back	200 mg	Some improvement
Yazzie Eq	8	Tendons	1 gm	Improved
Poodle	12	Kidneys, back	200 mg	Improved
Basset Hound	10	Back pain	200 mg	"much better"

Chapter Two

The Many Uses of Velvet Antler in the Practice of Medicine.

Mediating Tissue Regeneration.

We are constantly in search of natural substances which can aid us in our quest to promote healing of disease and trauma. Many therapies have presented themselves over the course of the past three decades, and velvet antler is one of them. Stem cells function to replenish dead or lost cells in areas of the body as needed. This could occur in the organ where the stem cell resides or in other organs. For example, bone marrow stem cells (also referred to as hematopoietic stem cells) would be able to replenish lost blood, and provide new immune cells during infection. At the same time, these stem cells have the capacity to detect damaged organs and migrate to repair the injured tissues. It is suspected neural stem cells may play a role in brain repair following injury and also in the replacement of dying neurons (brain cells). These subjects are the focus of active research in labs around the world. Scientists are speculating that certain nutrients could play important roles in maintaining the healthy renewal of replacement stem cells in the brain, blood, and other tissues. It may be possible, according to these scientists, to use certain nutrient combinations in the treatment of conditions that warrant stem cell replacement.

As organs that grow very quickly (up to 2.75 cm per day), velvet antler has been considered to be a source of factors mediating tissue regeneration. However, the nature of the factors responsible for the medicinal effects ascribed to it remained unclear. Recently, growing interest in "natural" or complementary medicine has encouraged research on the antlers themselves. This resulted in a demonstration of a number of growth factors expressed in the growing antlers, such as insulin-like growth factors (IGF)-1 and -2, transforming growth factor b (TFGb), epidermal growth factor, bone morphogenetic protein-4, neurotrophin-3, fibroblast growth factor-2, vascular endothelial growth factor, and nerve growth factor.

These factors may be responsible for the regenerative effects of antler preparations observed in animal or in vitro models and some of them are known players in immune responses. Endothelial Growth Factor (EGF), promotes healthy tissue development while also impeding abnormal growth, and promotes mesenchymal (lymphatic), glial (nerve), and epithelial (skin) cell proliferation. Vascular Endothelial Growth Factor (VEGF) promotes venous, venule, artery, arteriole, and capillary health by providing the essential co-factors for repairing and restoring damaged vessels.

Fibroblast Growth Factor (FGF) contains at least 19 different types of growth factors, of which their prominent role is in the development of skeletal and nervous systems in mammals. FGF is also located in the central nervous system and in peripheral nerves with less prominent effects including the regulation of both pituitary and ovarian cell function. The effects of antler velvet on cell growth and repair have been investigated in several areas. For example, antler regeneration not only involves bone, but also nerve tissue as well, that can grow up to one cm/day, an exceptional rate of growth.

Velvet antler increases muscle strength and has very powerful neurotropic (nerve-strengthening) properties. Neurotrophin Growth Factor (NGF) Recent work shows velvet antler contains a powerful nerve growth factor neurotrophin-3. NGF works synergistically with growth factors to promote neurite and nerve survival and development. One of the most exciting uses for Insulin-like Growth Factor (IGF-1) is the repair of nerve damage that occurs in injury or illness. When a nerve is damaged in a limb, the connection to muscle tissue is dramatically impaired. As a result, there is a loss of movement and a subsequent wasting of the affected muscle tissue.

Recent laboratory experiments on IGF-1 have demonstrated a stimulation of the protective myelin sheath around nerves. In degenerative diseases like multiple sclerosis, or ALS (Lou Gehrig's disease), damage around the sheath, stops signals from being transmitted between the brain and nerves. IGF-1 has been found to regrow myelin sheaths according to University of Michigan scientists. Although several growth factors are currently being studied, IGF-1 appears to be most effective at inducing the growth of the sheath and preventing neuronal cell death. Scientists removed dorsal root nerves from newborn rats and grew them in a dish. They found that if they stimulated the conditions of diabetes in the dish and then applied the IGF-1, it normalized nerve function. In studies where nerve cells have been placed in culture tubes, IGF -1 has been shown to have remarkable growth effects on spinal cord motor neurons by increasing motor neuron activity in spinal cultures by 150 to 270 percent. In certain animal studies it had a direct effect in stimulating nerve axons of the spinal cord motor neurons to regenerate. It increased intramuscular nerve sprouting 10-fold when it was given to normal adult rats. IGF-1 by itself or in combination with other growth factors could potentially stimulate nerve regeneration.[2]

The implications of these early studies are absolutely enormous! If IGF-1 can regenerate spinal cord motor neurons, it may be useful in treating devastating, fatal diseases like amyotrophic lateral sclerosis. And, one might speculate that it could be of value in conditions such as Degenerative Myelopathy.[3] One of the most exciting uses for IGF-1 is in repair of nerve damage that occurs in injury or illness. These nerves can regenerate to some extent. Severe damage of more than one-half inch may result in permanent injury. However, IGF-1 has repaired and reconnected severed nerve endings up to a distance of six millimeters. This has never, heretofore, been done. This may explain part of deer antler's ability to regenerate nerve tissue in deer.[4] In studies from Japan, deer velvet extract has shown to speed up the healing of damaged nerve tissue, and also to aid in the recovery of patients suffering from cervical and whiplash injuries.[5]

Deer Velvet and Anemias

Deer velvet has been shown to improve blood cell production, an advantage in many secondary anemias. It is "often used to increase blood counts, particularly in cases of anemia induced by chemotherapy," says TCM practitioner David Scrimgeour, LAc. "Velvet antler is very fast-growing, thus the association with it being able to quickly reproduce something like red blood cells."

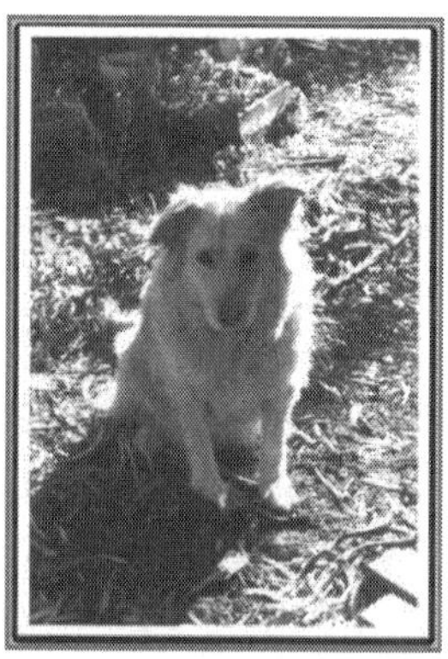

Case study: Freak was a two year old, 20 kg, mixed breed intact male. Freak had been found two days before he was brought to the medical pet clinic. Freak was emaciated, not eating well, and moved with difficulty. A complete physical examination revealed a temperature of 39.50C, pale mucus membranes, tachypnea and enlarged peripheral lymph nodes. At that stage, a Complete Blood Count was done. A blood smear showed non regenerative anemia, and a large number of highly active Monocytes and Morulae in the monocytes. Freak was diagnosed with chronic Ehrlichiosis and severe bone marrow depression.

Treatment: The owner was informed about the poor prognosis. Doxycycline 10 mg/kg SID was administered for 16 days along with bioactive deer velvet, 1500 mg per day.

Name of Dog: Freak				
Parameter	Normal Range	Day 1	Day 10	Day 30
Hematocrit	37.0 – 55.0	10.3	17.8	23.1
RBC	5.50 – 8.50	1.41	2.34	5.85
Hemoglobin	12.0 – 18.0	3.9	6.4	8.3
Platelets	175 - 500	62	40	98
WBC	5.50 – 16.90	1.85	3.64	6.6
Neurophil	2.00 – 12.00	1.3	2.64	4.37
Lymphocyte	0.50 – 4.90	0.15	0.56	1.39
Eosinophil	0.10 – 1.49	0.03	0.09	0.41
Monocyte	0.30 – 2.00	0.09	0.31	0.41
Basophil	0.00 – 0.10	0.0	0.04	0.03

Results: After two days the owner reported that Freak was much better, eating well and was playful. Hematology revealed remarkable improvement. The treatment for Ehrlichia was straight forward, but the rapid recovery was very impressive given the severity of the anemia. There were ups and downs as time progressed, as evidenced by the follow up blood tests. But, ten months after admission. Freak stabilized and was doing well. We believe that the bioactive deer velvet made a difference in the fast recovery from anemia.

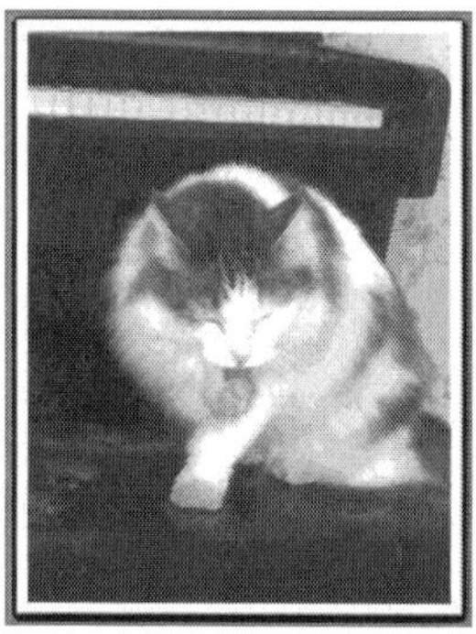

Case study: Rolly was a four-year-old domestic, long-haired, neutered male cat brought to the medical pet clinic with the complaints that he was not eating, and was less active than usual. His litter box was dry. He was mainly an indoor cat but would also go outside of the house. Rolly was fully vaccinated and ate dry commercial cat food. A complete clinical examination revealed very pale yellow mucous membranes and a distended bladder. At that stage, hematology and chemistry blood tests were carried out. On a blood smear, clinicians identified Mycoplasma hemofelis, spherocytes, reticlucytes and nucleated RBCs.

Diagnosis: Feline Infectious Anemia (mycoplasma hemofelis), regenerative anemia + secondary AIHA.

Treatment: Due to financial difficulties, no blood transfusion was carried out. Treatment consisted of Doxycycline at 40 mg P/O SID, Prednisone 8 mg IM, BID for seven days and then reduced to 1 mg/kg BID for seven days. Cimetedine BID, and Bioactive Deer velvet, 560 mg P/O SID, fluids, and Duphalyte (Nutrient solution-Pfizer).

Parameter	Normal Range	Day 1	Day 3	Day 7
Hematocrit	37.0 – 55.0	10.8	13.4	26.8
RBC	5.50 – 8.50	2.1	3.8	7.2
Hemoglobin	12.0 – 18.0	3.8	6.1	12.8
Platelets	175 - 500	400	400	400
WBC	5.50 – 16.90	13.3	3.9	6.29
Neurophil	2.00 – 12.00	5.35	2.76	3.10
Lymphocyte	0.50 – 4.90	5.25	0.7	2.15
Eosinophil	0.10 – 1.49	0.26	0.37	0.35
Monocyte	0.30 – 2.00	0.16	0.10	0.64
Basophil	0.00 – 0.10	0.05	0.03	0.06

Results: After twenty-four hours, Rolly started eating and blood tests were obtained after three and seven days respectively.

Immuno-modulation.

Velvet antler contains antibiotic-like Velvatin nucleotides. Velvet contains some hormonal components that can act as immunomodulators. It is known that estrogens regulate thymus function and suppress cell-mediated immune reactions. Antibody response and natural immunity (NK cytotoxicity, phagocytosis) are augmented by estradiol. Many of the immunological effects of testosterone are due to its conversion to estradiol by aromatase in the thymus and in other lymphoid organs. Research has also shown that in laboratory animals, velvet antler may prevent stress-stimulated hypertrophy of the adrenals and involution of the thymus.

Researchers in New Zealand investigated velvet antler's effect on human white blood cells, because of its long history of being taken for immune system support. Studies demonstrated that aqueous extracts of velvet antler were highly potent in causing an increase in human white blood cell count, particularly Monocytes. Monocytes represent three to seven percent of leukocytes in blood and are necessary to the immune function of lymph, spleen, bone marrow, and loose connective tissue. A recent study on bioactive deer velvet revealed several intriguing peptide sequences, similar to Bovine Hemoglobin peptide that can have antimicrobial properties.

After analysis of eight New Zealand red deer extracts,[6] it was determined that extracts had significant immune stimulant activity. The studies of the eight extracts used two dosage ranges. The investigators found that all extracts in the first set of dilutions carried some immune stimulant capacity. Those in the second set did as well, even in dilutions as low as 15mg/ml. It is postulated that due to cytokines in the antlers, the response is humoral, involving antibody stimulation, as opposed to being a cell-mediated response. And because of the potential for side effects pursuant to the use of any drug or supplement, it was significant to determine that even at the lowest dilution, immune enhancement was still observed.

Reduces Wound Healing Time

Research has shown that long standing wounds and ulcers also respond well to the growth hormone precursors in velvet antler and they have been suggested as factors in healing wounds, mending bones and helping with arthritic complaints. Deer velvet antler has been found to have extreme anabolic properties and could stimulate repair of tissue trauma after intensive exercise and post injury. The cartilaginous substance contains N-Acetyl Glucosamine that has been demonstrated to promote wound healing. In a 2008 study that examined the effects of deer antler extract on healing wounds in rats, researchers found that deer antlers appeared to help "stimulate and accelerate the repair of cutaneous wounds"[7]. Scientists looked at how the rats' wounds were affected by applying ointment made from deer antlers. The results are pretty stunning. The photos below show the healing rate comparison with and without velvet antler. The sample on the top is "Day 0" and the sample on the bottom is "Day 7".

Without Velvet Antler

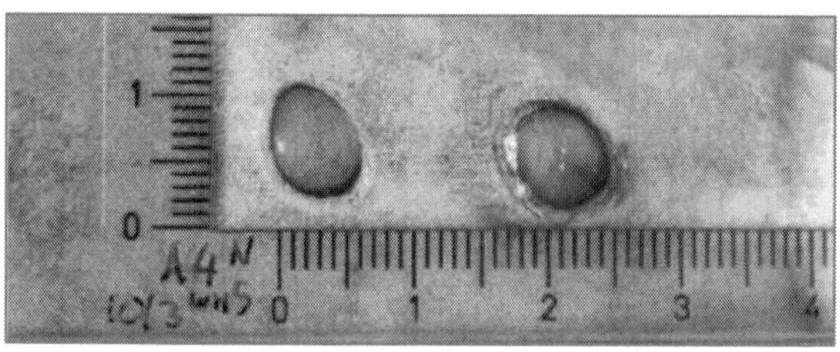

With Velvet Antler

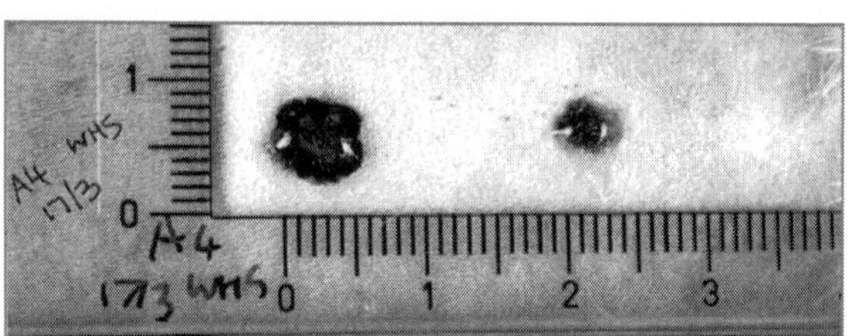

Researchers write, "In addition, the wound treated with a high concentration antler ointment, and the control closed completely at post-injury day 40, day 44 and day 60, respectively." This means that wounds treated with deer antler appeared to heal at a faster rate than those that weren't.

Dermatology –

Atopy, Alopecias, and Black Skin Disease.

Allergies and atopy typically appear between one and three years of age. There is a genetic predisposition, and a progressive worsening is typical. Dogs with atopic dermatitis often have concurrent allergies and are prone to relapsing skin and ear infections, and anal sacculitis. In the case of an allergic inflammatory phase, pollen or other protein motifs trigger the degranulation of the mast cell. This releases histamin and heparin, which causes vasodilation and permeability of the vascular wall, along with dilution of the blood. Thereby, this results in swelling and increased fluid secretion as the body attempts to liquefy and eliminate the invading antigens. Both local and central control mechanisms come to play in the body's attempt to regulate this cycle of activity and promote the reparatory processes.

Factors to consider in allergies include:

- Skin (atopic dermatitis)
- Mucous membranes (allergic rhinitis, asthma)
- Liver overload
- Matrix toxicity
- So-called mucosal distress

There is a large body of anecdotal evidence that has studied the use of deer velvet for conditions such as psoriasis in humans. Having been apprised of some raging successes in humans, we have put a number of dogs and cats on a product which contains bioactive deer velvet, perna, colostrum, zinc, and porphyra (Red algae). With few exceptions, we have had some remarkably improved dermatological cases. (Several humans that I know personally, have benefited greatly from this or a similar supplement.)

Alopecia X.

The cause of this alopecic (hair loss) condition in dogs is unclear, but several theories have been proposed. These include abnormal adrenal steroidogenesis, growth hormone deficiency, an adrenal sex hormone imbalance, or even excessive production of androgenic steroids by the adrenal glands. Current theories suggest that a local follicular receptor dysregulation may be the underlying disorder. The condition is uncommon but the average incidence is in dogs two to five years old.

Chow Chows, Pomeranians, Keeshonds, Samoyeds, Alaskan malamutes, Siberian huskies, and miniature poodles are predisposed. Gradual bilateral loss of primary hairs progresses to complete alopecia of the neck, tail, caudodorsum, perineum, and caudal thighs. The loss then eventually becomes generalized over the trunk, but the head and front limbs are spared, so they resemble little lions. The alopecic skin may become hyperpigmented, thin, and hypotonic. Mild secondary seborrhea and superficial pyoderma may occur. Affected dogs are otherwise quite well without systemic signs.

Fluffy – Bald Pomeranian

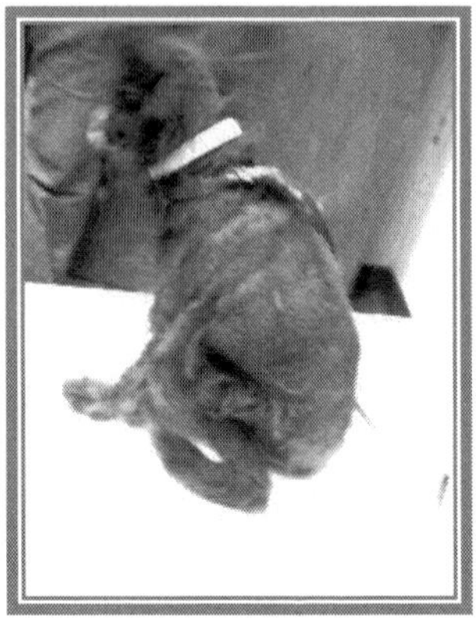

Condition: Chronic alopecia, stubborn refractory ringworm.

Treatment: Administered PentaGenesis (velvet antler) and Blue Green Algae combination.

Result: Regrew coat, but lost it again, after discontinuing therapy. Put back on supplements. Condition stable for several years to date.

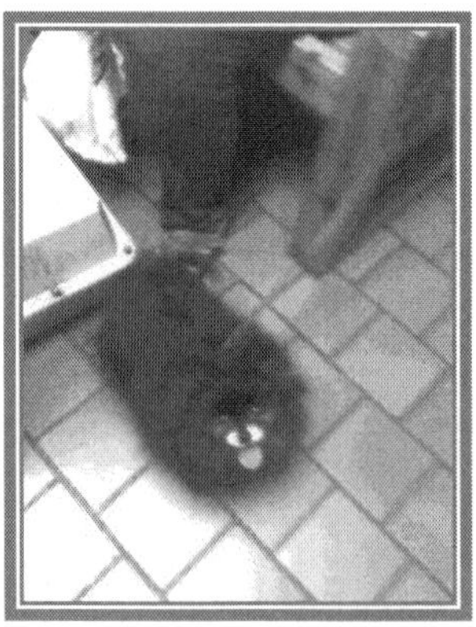

Tiki – Keeshond

Condition: Generalized alopecia three years in duration. All bloodwork and diagnostics were within normal limits, non-definitive.

Treatment: Given PentaGenesis (velvet antler) 2 tablets daily, starting in December 2013. Photo to right: Hair re-growing slowly April 2014.

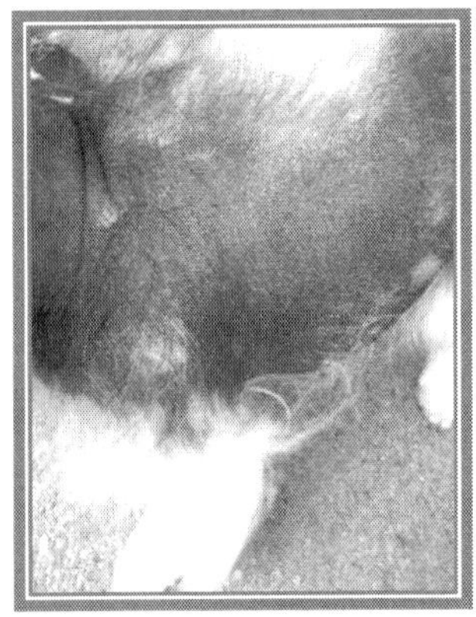

* Increased dosage to three PentaGenesis daily In July 2014.

August 2014:

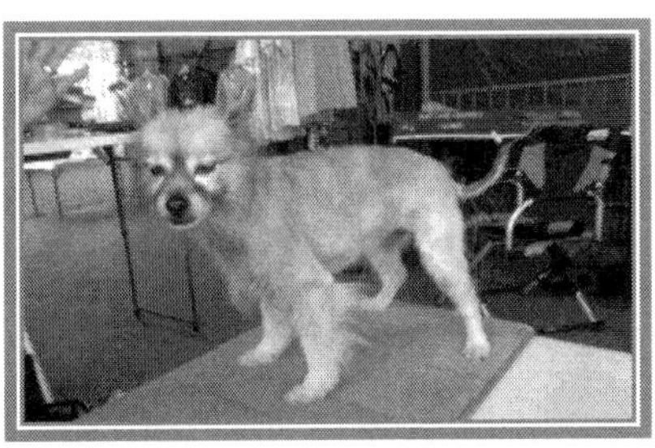

November 2014:

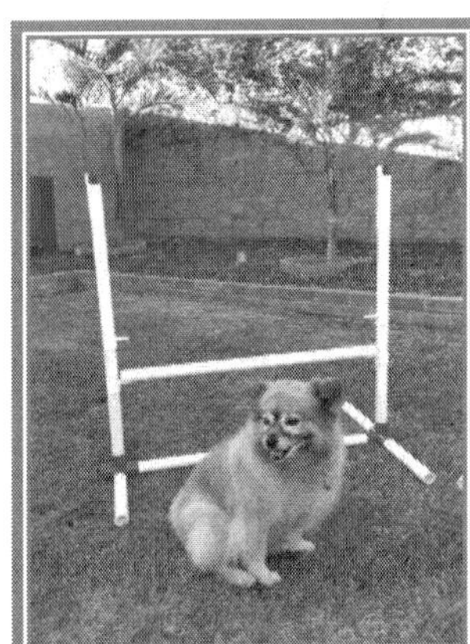

Chapter Three

Pharmacology of Velvet Antler

Antlers grow by endochondral ossification. This is the same way that long bones grow. A major non-collagenous protein, proteoglycan, is a protein substituted with glycosaminoglycan chains. This protein occurs in the cartilaginous tissue of antler. While its use in the antler is not understood, it has been shown that proteoglycan in cartilage, also called aggrecan, regulates differentiation of chondrocytes and may also control calcium concentration in the growth plates where endochondral ossification occurs. Immunohistochemical techniques have isolated decorin, a proteoglycan, in wapiti antler, which has a glucuronate-rich glycosaminoglycan chain.[8]

The history of antler as a medicinal substance stretches back thousands of years. Although the most well-documented ancient uses come from China and the Far East, other cultures from Northern Europe and Northern Asia to North American and ancient Rome have also benefited from the use of antler as a tonic and for treatment of a variety of medical conditions.

These include:

- Joint pain
- Kidney and liver problems
- Stomach ulcers
- Gout
- Headaches
- Eczema
- Low energy
- Chills

Even today, antler extract compounds are listed in the pharmacopoeia of the former USSR Health Ministry as "tonic drugs." In clinical studies, New Zealand scientists at AgResearch Invermay, near Dunedin, have shown that velvet can stimulate or can down-regulate the body's immune system. Research showed that treating human white blood cells with extracts of New Zealand velvet stimulated the immune system, as measured by increased production of white blood cells. This response – immune-potentiation in scientific terms – is the body's defense mechanism. Increased numbers of white blood cells are produced to fight "intruder" bugs. Velvet antler is a homeostatic enabler, and effective bio-regulator that makes the immune system more balanced. As mentioned previously velvet antler is composed of a variety of different tissues, including cartilage. It is also rich in collagen, a crucial protein, and glycosaminoglycans.

New Zealand velvet contains nearly forty key bioactive compounds, including:

- *Hyaluronic acid* is the cement of connective tissue and a component of synovial fluid that lubricates joints.
- *Glycosaminoglycans* (GAGs)
- *Chondroitin sulfate*, a carbohydrate that attracts fluid into proteoglycan molecules and protects cartilage from destructive enzymes.
- *Glucosamine sulfate*, the building block of proteoglycans, which are important for the elasticity of joints and the structure of joint cartilage, and a reported anti-inflammatory that is easily absorbed by the body.
- *Glycosphingolipids* are involved with cell metabolism and the cells of the nervous system; Amino acids - essential proteins.
- *Collagen* is a major structural protein that gives strength to skin, cartilage, bones and other connective tissue.

- *Essential fatty acids* including Omega 3 & 6 are natural anti-inflammatories that build cells and boost energy.
- *Minerals & trace elements* including: Calcium (CA), Copper (Cu), Iron (FE), Manganese (Mn), Selenium (SE), Magnesium (Mg), Potassium (K), Phosphorus (P), Sulphur (S), Zinc (Zn).
- *Monoamine-oxidase inhibitors* enhance mood
- *Prostaglandins* are powerful anti-inflammatory agents.
- *Phosphorus* helps build bones and teeth, and is a key component of metabolic reaction
- *Polysaccharides* help regulate blood clotting activity.
- *All essential amino acids* are the building blocks of protein.
- *Growth factors* aid in cartilage cell development.

Chapter Four

Velvet Antler for Osteoarthritis – A potential alternative to drugs or surgery.

Therapies based on New Zealand velvet antler can provide a natural, holistic treatment to help relieve symptoms associated with joint problems caused by osteoarthritis in pets. As well as providing relief from pain and inflammation and increasing mobility, velvet antler provides other long-term benefits for their general well-being. With the exception of expensive surgery for joint replacement, there is no cure for osteoarthritis in pets. Non-steroidal anti-inflammatory drugs are commonly used. They can be very effective but like all drugs they carry risks of side effects. Velvet antler has been shown to be an effective alternative by a number of veterinarians practicing a holistic approach to small animal treatment.

According to Dr. Doron Zur, Animals Kapiti Ltd, New Zealand, "Eighty-five percent of my clients, whose dogs and cats used a supplement containing velvet antler and green lipped mussel, found that there was a marked improvement in the agility and mobility of their pets.

There was also a noticeable improvement in the condition of the animal's coats and skin. Velvet Antler proved to be a suitable alternative treatment to the NSAID products with the added bonus that no negative side effects were noted."

All veterinarians are schooled in the treatment of osteoarthritis as caused by the loss of cartilage in bone joints. We learn that in normal joints, cartilage serves as a buffer between bones. Usually the body replenishes cartilage as it wears away, but in the case of osteoarthritis, cartilage deteriorates faster than the body can replace it causing the bones to rub together, resulting in pain, swelling and loss of joint mobility. This can be a result of abnormalities like hip dysplasia, from trauma, or just from the wear and tear of an active lifestyle. Excess weight, poor nutrition and joint trauma can make the condition worse.

Osteoarthritis (OA) is a painful musculoskeletal condition in dogs. It is often secondary to structural abnormalities, such as hip or elbow dysplasia or ligament injury. Most treatments for osteoarthritis attempt to reduce pain and maintain joint function, but these treatments do little to restore joint health. Many prescription and over-the-counter non-steroidal anti-inflammatory drugs actually prevent the growth of collagen in joints, causing further cartilage degeneration. These drugs can also produce other serious side effects such as deterioration of the gastrointestinal tract lining, and liver and kidney damage.

Research has led to the development of a broad range of pharmaceutical approaches to alleviate clinical signs by acting on the degenerative process, the associated inflammatory process, or both. Deer velvet antler is a well-known medicament in the Chinese materia medica, and has been used clinically in East Asia for thousands of years in the treatment of various diseases and as a tonic.

This traditional Chinese medicine is a nutritional supplement made from the inner core of deer antler in the velvet stage of growth. Observations from in vivo studies[9] demonstrated an anti-inflammatory effect of a peptide (pilose antler peptide) isolated from velvet antler in a rodent model of inflammation.[10] These studies, combined with the knowledge that chondroitin sulfate is found in velvet antler, suggested that this material could be useful in the treatment of OA. Researchers believe that the imbalance between cartilage erosion and regeneration in osteoarthritis suffers, is caused by a lack of glycosaminoglycans which play a vital role in the structural integrity of cartilage. Several studies indicate that velvet antler can reduce or even eliminate symptoms associated with osteoarthritis. Recent clinical tests suggest oral ingestion of glycosaminoglycan-peptide complex, or components such as chondroitin sulfate and glucosamine sulfate – both found in velvet antler – may help stimulate cartilage repair. Placebo-controlled double-blind studies of both humans and animals on the therapeutic effects of glycosaminoglycan-peptide complex appear to confirm these investigations.

Chondroitin sulfate, the most abundant glycosaminoglycan found in velvet antler, is used in surgery to stabilize tissue. Studies on humans indicate regular oral ingestion of chondroitin sulfate can significantly reduce the symptoms associated with osteoarthritis. The compound appears to inhibit enzymes that deplete cartilage nutrition. Chondroitin sulfate molecules are long chains of sugars and sulfur that create tiny spaces filled with fluid. These spaces protect and cushion joints. Randomized studies of glucosamine indicate the compound not only inhibits cartilage degradation but also helps repair damaged cartilage.

An eight-week double-blind trial of glucosamine on forty osteoarthritis sufferers found that the compound had significantly longer-lasting benefits than the commonly prescribed pain killer ibuprofen. Other studies indicate that the effects appear to continue as long as six to twelve weeks after subjects stop taking glucosamine.

"An uncontrolled trial on dogs with arthritis was carried out using placebos and velvet antler, and found a positive response in 84 percent of the velvet antler group and no response in the placebo group. The velvet Antler supplement appeared to increase the activity levels of all dogs, some of them exhibiting behaviors of their youth such as ball catching, jumping up in the car etc."- *Mr. E. van Schreven, Veterinarian, South Canterbury, New Zealand*

"When introduced to velvet antler, at first I was very skeptical but I decided to use it on a dog that had not responded to any other (conventional) treatment. Within only a few days the dog had started running! After that, velvet antler became very popular among my colleague vets in my practices, and we have now prescribed several hundred bottles of velvet antler tablets. Furthermore, I am now using V-One, (a human velvet antler product) myself." *-Dr. Amiel Shlomi, Northern Israel*

"From a medical point of view velvet antler has shown a very positive effect on fracture healing, arthritis therapy, surgery recovery and overall wellness, including improved energy and vitality. Anyone who truly cares about their pets will give them velvet antler – it ensures the animals will live a healthier, happier and pain-free life". *-Dr. DeGrofft, DVM Loveland, Colorado, USA*

Chapter Five

Clinical Trials and Research

Trials on Osteoarthritis

Particular chronic degenerative conditions such as osteoarthritis (OA) and rheumatoid arthritis (RA), are attributed to alterations in collagen synthesis, changes in cellular metabolism, changes in endogenous cellular environments which inhibit production of type II collagen, or to the collagen itself as a contributor to the degeneration. In RA the synovial membranes of multiple joints are inflamed; fibroblasts in the synovium invade and damage both cartilage and bone.

Oral tolerance models have been used as a method of creating antigen specific tolerance in autoimmune diseases such as multiple sclerosis and uveitis. This parallels allergic desensitization when the patient, little by little, through carefully controlled exposure becomes desensitized to the allergen until the reaction finally abates. As an autoantigen, type II collagen activates T-cells and also the chronic degeneration of joint cartilage of bones. In reaction to its oral administration, T-cells generated by the immune response contain cytokines that can suppress part of the degenerative response that occurs in RA. Velvet antler is a significant source of type II collagen and worthy of serious consideration in the treatment of RA.

>Clinical evaluation of a powder of quality deer velvet antler for the treatment of osteoarthrosis in dogs. - Moreau M, Dupuis J, Bonneau NH, Lécuyer M; Can Vet J. 2004 Feb;45(2):133-9.

Abstract

A powder of quality deer velvet antler (QEVA) was evaluated on client-owned dogs with osteoarthrosis (OA) in a clinical, double-blind, and placebo-controlled study. Thirteen dogs received a placebo for 30 days and then QEVA for 60 days. Twenty-five other dogs received QEVA for 60 days. Gait analysis measured with a force plate, clinical signs assessed by an orthopedic surgeon, performances in daily life activities and vitality assessed by the owners, and complete blood analyses' were obtained at days 0, after 30 days of placebo and/or 60 days of QEVA. On placebo, the thirteen dogs did not show significant improvement ($P < 0.05$). However, the gait of the 13 study dogs, their performances in daily life activities, and their vitality were significantly improved on QEVA. These were based on changes in values exceeding those observed when placebo was administered. The twenty-five dogs on QEVA for sixty days showed similar improvements. No clinical changes were revealed on blood analyses. Administration of QEVA was effective in alleviating the condition in arthritic dogs.

The beneficial effects of QEVA on arthritic dogs were objectively and subjectively demonstrated in this study. Based on the improvements observed here, consideration should be given to a powder of quality deer velvet antler in the treatment of canine OA. Further fundamental investigation in OA cartilage explants to evaluate the capacity of QEVA to reduce or inhibit the degenerative process would be interesting. Also, the long-term safety of administering QEVA needs to be investigated, as does the magnitude of improvement with a well-defined and frequently prescribed OA medication on dogs afflicted with osteoarthrosis.

"I conducted five separate trials on patients that were already being medicated with preparations to assist them with their mobility. We did not achieve a 100 percent positive response to the use of velvet antler. However, I became hooked on the usefulness of this dietary supplement, and thus committed to become more involved in its mystic mechanisms and uses. After all is said, it is the patient (dog's) response and their owner's complete joy in the visual benefits that has cemented my belief in this product*".- Mr. G. Baitz (BVSc) MRCVS MASFM Esther, United Kingdom*

Velvet Antler (VA) Research Overview

Velvet antler demonstrates an ability to prevent or reduce both shock and stress responses. Rats given velvet antler prior to exposure to extreme temperatures and to electric shock demonstrated quicker recovery times than those that did not receive antler treatment.[11]

Tests also show that in laboratory animals, velvet antler may prevent stress-stimulated hypertrophy of the adrenal glands and involution of the thymus.[12]

Tip section preparations have also been observed to stimulate wound healing.[13] Erythropoiesis, increased red blood cell production, has been observed in anemic rats and rabbits given velvet antler products; this finding supports the empirical use of velvet antler for conditions of anemia in humans.[14]

Velvet extracts also slows tumor growth and demonstrated antitumor activity against Bacillus P-92, a tumor cell line, in mice.[15] Fermented velvet antler increases the survival rate of mice that have tumors from 25-40 percent.[16]

Miscellaneous Research

1) *Effects on growth rate and fetal development*: Feeding antler diet for fifty-four days showed a significant effect on the growth rate of immunized rats. VA powder resulted in a significant increase of HDL-C/LDL-C ratio, which suggests cardioprotection. Unknown factors from the antler may be useful for the prevention of the risk of coronary heart disease. Hematocrit value and iron content in plasma also significantly increased by feeding antler powder.[17] Another study showed that supplementation of powdered velvet antler resulted in improved growth, feed efficiency and development of some intestinal organs in growing and adult rats.[18] VA as a supplement, given to female rats during gestation,

improved both physical and neurological development of offspring.[19]

2) *Cardioprotection*: Japanese Studies at the Oriental Medicine Research Center of the Kitasato Institute, Tokyo, Japan, have identified polysaccharides that tend to reduce the clotting tendency of blood, and have a blood thinning effect. This can contribute to improved circulation, reduced stroke risk and improved cardiovascular health without the attendant side effects of currently popular drugs.[20] An intriguing study reported in 2013, showed cardiac repair with supplementation of antler velvet in rats, following heart failure subsequent to myocardial infarction.[21]

3) *Tissue Repair and Wound Healing*: Deer velvet grows at up to 2cm per day, and all support tissues, including blood vessels, must also grow at that rate. It is possible that VA possesses unique factors which can allow blood vessels to grow that fast. VA has been shown to increase the number of blood vessels in fertilized chicken eggs, and show increased filamentous threads of blood vessels in tissue culture. There are likely to be therapeutic properties, for example in tissue repair and wound healing.[22] Velvet Antler Extract (VAE) may lead the

fibroblasts towards the activated status that can be seen in the wound healing process, and this raises the possibility of therapeutically using VAE for fast wound closure.[23]

4) *Liver protection*: VA may contain a liver protecting factor, and recent data shows that for 2 liver enzymes, AST and ALT, levels were lower, an indication of less damage – in animals fed deer velvet compared to the controls.[24]

5) *Repair of bone*: In one study, VA polypeptides promoted proliferation of chondrocytes and osteoblast precursors, and fracture healing in a rat study. The healing rate in a velvet antler total polypeptides (VATP) treated group was higher (75%) than that of control group (25%). In another study, cells in regenerating deer antler cartilage provide a microenvironment that supports osteoclast differentiation. Velvet antler polypeptides promote proliferation of chondrocytes and osteoblast precursors and fracture healing.[25]

6) *Performance and endurance*: VA test subjects showed a shorter recovery time between exercises and were able to support an increased work load. An increase in heart strength and blood volume pumping, a significant reduction in blood pressure, and a decrease in cholesterol

levels have been demonstrated. VA can increase performance and endurance. In studies of anabolic agents and their effects on muscle composition, endurance and strength, VA has been shown to help increase muscle restoration following exertion.[26]

7) *Liver and kidney*: Due to its androgenic activity, VA was used to determine its effects on the liver and kidney. Liver tissue damaged with chloroform was able to recover following VA treatment. In follow-up studies it was observed that protein formation in both the liver and kidney was enhanced. This was due to effects of VA on RNA polymerase activity.[27]

8) *Anti-Allergy, Anti-Asthma*: VA has been shown to reduce allergic symptoms and asthma in a mouse study via regulation of the Th1/Th2 balance, with reduction of eosinophilia, IgE, and pro-inflammatory cytokines. This was a dose dependent reduction, and lends credence to clinical reports of improved lung function.[28]

9) *Immune support*: VA treated lab animals showed an increase in monocytes, increased neutrophils, enhanced phagocytosis and immunoglobulin levels, all necessary to immune function. Being a skin derivative, VA contains melanin, the major pigment in the skin, which may

quench reactive oxygen species, thus reducing oxidative stress and apoptosis. Melanin has been reported as an activator of T-cell responses and may be important in pathogenesis of autoimmune diseases such as uveitis and vitiligo. VA has been shown to increase T-cell proliferation and cell division in a dose-dependent manner. There was concern that VA extract could increase the risk of T-cell malignancies by inducing proliferation of T-cells. However, studies show that VA extract co-stimulates proliferation of both CD4+ and CD8+ T cells, but not T cell lymphoma. VA can be described as regulatory rather than stimulatory, as it tends to balance the immune response.[29]

10) *Diabetes*: VA as a supplement, can be of value in diabetes not only for its ability to help repair neurological damage, but as a blood sugar regulator by normalizing diabetic processes in the gangliosides.[30]

11) *Post surgery recovery*: VA has been shown to improve the rate of recovery after surgical interventions. The rate of wound healing is one contributory factor, but there are many other components of recovery that can be addressed by VA.[31]

12) *Anti-ulcer, anti-inflammatory*: VA polysaccharides have been associated with antiulcer effects. Polysac-

charides in VA may be responsible for the anti-inflammatory actions in the treatment of mammary hyperplasia. Sulfated polysaccharides have diverse functions in the tissues from which they originate, as we have noted from our discussion of Porphyra and Perna. They can bind with proteins at several levels of specificity and are involved mainly in the development, cell differentiation, cell adhesion, cell signaling and cell matrix interactions. These bioactive molecules present a great potential for medical, pharmaceutical and biotechnological applications such as wound dressings, biomaterials, tissue regeneration and 3D culture scaffolds and even drugs.[32]

13) E*strogen replacement therapy*: Since epidermal growth factor supplants estrogen in genital tract development, it also may be useful in the estrogen replacement therapies.[33] With its traditional role in lower body weakness, it would be intriguing to study whether this supplement could improve estrogen dependent incontinence in dogs. This has become much more common in recent decades. IGF- I, luteinizing hormones and prostaglandins, alter inflammatory events, muscular atrophy and androgen formation.

14) *Wound healing*: In addition, studies suggest that peptide growth factors, such as epidermal growth factor (EGF), has a role in wound healing. Topical treatment with a water-soluble VA extract accelerates repair of cutaneous wounds in streptozotocin-induced diabetic rats.[34]

15) *Anemia*: VA, as an erythropoeitic agent, can normalize blood cell counts without the need for iron supplements. Anemia was induced in rabbits by a single injection of a chemical agent. When the anemia was most severe, they were treated with aqueous deer velvet extracts. All deer velvet extracts studied sped up recovery from anemia and raised erythrocyte number, hemoglobin, iron, and packed volume over the resting level.[35]

Clinical Evaluation of Bioactive New Zealand Deer Velvet (BADV) to Speed up the Recovery from Anemia"[36] Trial done on 13 Healthy dogs of both sexes with average weight of 55-70 pounds. There ages ranged from two to five years. 450 ml blood was drawn on Day 0. HCT was run on Day 0, 1, 4, and 7. Four dogs received a placebo. Nine dogs were treated with 1500 mg BADV BID. (see chart next page)

B.A.D.V

Parameters	Normal Range	Day 0	Day 1	Day 4	Day 7
HTC	37.0 - 55.0	44.1 +/- 5	33 +/- 2.5	40.3 +/- 3	46.3 +/- 5
RBC	5.50 - 8.50	6.47 +/- 1	4.83 +/- 1	5.93 +/- 1.2	6.6 +/- 1.5
HGB	12.0 - 18.0	14.8 +/- 1	12.6 +/- 0.8	13.43 +/- 0.5	14.57 +/- 1

Placebo

Parameters	Normal Range	Day 0	Day 1	Day 4	Day 7
HTC	37.0 - 55.0	44.2 +/- 4	33.5 +/- 2.2	32.2 +/- 2	36.1 +/- 2
RBC	5.50 - 8.50	6.49 +/- 1.1	4.90 +/- 1	4.8 +/- 1	5.7 +/- 2
HGB	12.0 - 18.0	14.85 +/- 0.9	12.1 +/- 1.1	13 +/- 1	13.2 +/- 1

Results: Dogs that received BADV recovered from the anemia much faster than the dogs that received the placebo. Dogs that received BADV showed an increase in hematocrit level and RBC after day 4, compared to the dogs that received the placebo. Dogs that received BADV were back to the original hematocrit level and RBC in 7 days. The dogs that received the placebo, on the other hand, were back to the original hematocrit level only after 14 days.

Chapter Six

Velvet Antler - A Word about Cancer

Velvet antler (VA) has been scrutinized as a pro-neoplastic substance, primarily because of its angiogenesis potential. The question often comes up, so it is worth addressing.

A benefit of velvet antler according the principles of traditional Chinese medicine (TCM) is that it can stimulate the Yang and is used for conditions of Yang deficiencies. Ben-Xiang Wang at the Proceedings of the 1996 International Symposium on Deer Science and Deer Products described studies showing he performed where the treatment of rats with a velvet antler extract resulted in marked increases in the numbers of monocytes, suggesting the presence of components that might affect the immune system.[37]

VA has been found to be highly effective in increasing white blood cell counts and defending against leukemia cells.[38] Almost 250 papers have been published since 1930 on the manufacture, composition and biochemical effect of deer antler velvet extract. Results consistently showed benefits in number of areas. Scientific studies by Dr. Peter Fennessy of the Invermay Research Center in Otago, New Zealand revealed high amounts of Insulin-like Growth Factor-1, or IGF-1, which is known to promote cell growth. However, Dr Fennessy also found anti-tumor and anti-viral effects, in his studies.[39]

In New Zealand, researchers have found that extracts from velvet antler have reduced tumor cell growth (Suttie et al. 1994) which may show them to be useful in the fight against cancer. Anti-tumor activity of antler and antler fermented in Bacillus P-92 were demonstrated in mice. The result showed that the amount of free amino acids, polypeptides and other compounds that produce healthful effects were more bioavailable. The survival rate of mice with tumors increased from twenty-five to forty percent. The neutrophil levels in the mice were increased two to three-fold for antler and three to four-fold for fermented antler, which increased the body's ability to resist injury and disease. Results suggest that fermentation increases some of the health benefits of velvet antler. While there is no evidence to date showing that deer velvet actually cures cancer, experiments carried out in Russia have shown extracts to increase survival rate and, in some cases, to inhibit the spread of tumor cells in rats and mice.[40]

In addition, a study conducted by the East-West Research Institute (Kyung Hee University, Korea) and the Korean Food and Drug Administration found that mice with tumors lost less weight and suffered lower levels of kidney damage than those treated with the frequently-prescribed anti-cancer drug cis-Platin (CDDP). Velvet antler also appeared to boost the effectiveness of CDDP when used in conjunction with the cancer drug. Those mice given a combination of antler extract and CDDP survived longer and had fewer side effects than mice given CDDP alone.[41]

To determine whether the extracts of New Zealand deer velvet are effective in anti-cancer treatments, AgResearch has been running clinical trials in Korea and according to Dr. Joseph Mark Suttie, MBBS BSc, the first series of experiments have shown positive results. Transforming Growth Factor Alpha is found many times in large amounts in tumors. This may cause the average reader alarm, thinking that TGF-A is in some way causing or is responsible for the tumor or cancer. The opposite is the case.

Transforming Growth Factor Beta is a protein that controls proliferation, cellular differentiation, and other functions in most cells. It plays a role in immunity, cancer, heart disease, diabetes, and Marfan syndrome. TGF-beta acts as an antiproliferative factor in normal epithelial cells and at early stages of oncogenesis.

Epidermal growth factor EGF is a ligand (a substance that binds with another molecule for a specific purpose). EGF binds to epidermal growth factor receptors (EGFR). Science has proven that without EGF, and to some extent another growth factor called transforming growth factor alpha (TFGa), epidermal growth factor receptors (EGFR) would cause an improper proliferation of certain epidermal cells that would result in tumor growth and cancer.

Insufficient EGFR signaling in humans is associated with the development of neurodegenerative diseases, such as multiple sclerosis and Alzheimer's disease. Studies have shown that in mice, loss of signaling by EGFR results in embryonic lethality with defects in organs including the lungs, skin, heart and brain. Excessive EGFR signaling is associated with the development of a wide variety of types of solid tumor. It is found in many human cancers and research shows that their excessive signaling may be critical factors in the development and malignancy of these tumors. As we continue to point out, a proper balance in all areas of the body (homeostasis), especially with hormones and growth factors, is the key to health and being devoid of disease and illness. Therefore, if you do research into the importance of Epidermal growth factor (EGF), you will discover clinical studies being done with EGF relating to the negative growth effects on certain carcinomas (cancers) as well as ulcerative colitis and other GI diseases.

European researchers have shown that growth hormone and IGF-1 do what antioxidants cannot do. IGF -1 initiates the transport of nucleic acids into the nucleus of the cell where the DNA resides. It gives the raw material needed to repair damage to the DNA and initiates cell division. Thus, IGF -1 actually repairs the blueprint of life and helps to retard the aging process. When the DNA is repaired it can better resist carcinogens and protect us from cancer. The question then arises, can it really reduce the incidence of cancer or does it promote cancer?

A major problem with the drugs used in chemotherapy is the damage they cause to the body while destroying the cancer cells. However, during experiments it was discovered that the aqueous extracts of deer velvet increased the effectiveness of the anti-cancer drugs while at the same time reducing their side effects. They were clearly potent at reducing the damaging side effects of the anti-cancer drug, in particular by reducing damage to the kidneys.[42]

Dr. James Suttie's team tested the effects of extract on human peripheral lymphocytes (white blood cells) in culture. They compared these results to those of human recombinant interleukin 2 (IL-2), which is a natural growth factor for T-lymphocytes. The team found that all concentrations, antler ages, and antler sections tested had a proliferative effect on the lymphocytes. As was the case for the anti-inflammatory and anti-cancer effects of antler. Age and section did affect the efficacy of the extract. The most potent immunopotentiation was seen in the upper part of antler harvested at eighty-five days. The effect of this extract was so strong that it approximated the results seen from IL-2.[43]

Deer velvet's protective effects are also apparent in the area of cancer research. A deer velvet preparation increased the survival rate of mice exposed to radiation.[44] Reports of enhancement of immune function from velvet antler demonstrate significant immune stimulatory activity from several preparations, as well as enhancement of phagocytes and immunoglobulin levels in mice. An increase in monocytes in rats, cells necessary to the immune function of lymph, spleen, bone marrow, and loose connective tissue also has been reported.[45]

Human Cancer Studies: The landmark study of cartilage therapy for cancer began with Dr. John Prudden in 1974 when he was granted a study protocol by the U.S. Food and Drug Administration. All patients enrolled, had failed with chemotherapy, radiation, and surgery, and multiple cancers were studied: breast, cervix, ovary, prostate, lung, liver, bone, stomach, pancreas, brain, thyroid, and Hodgkin's Disease (lymph).

Ninety percent of the patients had a positive response and some of the cures were achieved fastest when chemotherapy was combined with cartilage. In fact, cartilage protected the patients from the severe side effects of chemotherapy. Thus cartilage supplements can be taken with standard forms of treatment.

Dr Prudden and his contemporaries theorize that the mechanism of oral efficacy of cartilage is immune stimulation, because it closely resembles foetal mesenchyme.

This is tissue in its earliest stages of development, from which skin, fat, muscle, bone and bone marrow (a base our immune system) all evolve. Thus, the effect of mesenchyme on any tissue is potent normalization, and modulation of the immune system Dr. Prudden's study was conducted with bovine (calf) cartilage, but it appears the health benefits from cartilage is not species specific. Cartilage from cows, sharks, chickens, and now deer antler appears to have medicinal value.[46]

Chapter Seven

Velvet Antler. On the Cutting Edge – Stem Cell Research

Stem cells, with the capability to differentiate into varieties of cells, have been isolated from a number of tissues, including bone marrow, fat tissues, umbilical cord blood, placenta and menstrual blood. Recent research has focused on both pluripotent stem cells, (able to differentiate into all body cell types) and multipotent stem cells (able to differentiate into some specific cell types). Multipotent stem cells were identified early and have a longer history of studies.

Researchers are interested in deer velvet, because they are very peculiar organs, in that they are lost and regrown annually – a rare example of a completely regenerating organ in mammals. Deer antler has been subjected to differentiation assays for osteogenic (bone), adipogenic (fat) and chondrogenic (cartilage) lineages under culture conditions specific for each lineage to confirm the multilineage differentiation ability of antler multipotent stem cells. It was found that deer antler tissue might be a "valuable source of stem cells" that could be a potentially useful source of regenerative therapeutics in veterinary science.[47]

Researchers have sought to use transplanted stem cells for many regenerative purposes. Using them to regenerate neural cells following stroke or spinal-cord injuries, or using stem cells to help regenerate failing or injured organs. "We successfully isolated and characterized antler tissue-derived multipotent stem cells and confirmed that the isolated cells are self-renewing and can differentiate into multiple lineages," said study co-author Dr. Kyung-Sun Kang of the College of Veterinary Medicine at Seoul National University. "Using optimized culture conditions, deer antler displayed vigorous cell proliferation."[48] Stem cells in deer antler may, in the future, give us the ability to restore organs damaged through cancer, or excision, or trauma.

Conclusion

Velvet antler has been used safely and effectively with a variety of beneficial results for centuries by Russians and Orientals. It is known to be used for arthritis and rheumatic conditions that are sensitive to seasonal cold, damp weather, low energy, low sex drive, osteoporosis, hypothyroid and hypoadrenal conditions. Research has shown that VA is useful for the healing of wounds after surgery, broken bones, and could aid in trauma recovery. Its anabolic effects are important for reducing wasting and debilitation.

Antler regeneration not only involves bone, but nerve tissue as well, which can grow up to 1 cm/day, an exceptional rate of growth. The effect is thought to be due to increases in glycolosis, which is a necessary process in the maintenance of healthy nerve tissue. Oxygen metabolism, blood cell formation and muscle tissue enhancement may stimulate rejuvenative and tonic actions that benefit athletes, the elderly and cardiovascular disease patients alike. The nutrigenomic potential of deer velvet products is rather remarkable, and the burgeoning data from past and ongoing research make it a nutrient powerhouse to watch in the future.

Resource

In North America:

New Zealand Velvet Antler Products for Veterinarians.

(866)-897-5688 (Eastern time zone)

Website: www.NZDeerVelvetProducts.com

Email: info@nzdeervelvetproductsUSA.com

Index

adrenal, 22, 26, 27, 44
adrenals, 22
Allergies, 25, 26
alopecia, 7, 8, 25, 26, 27, 28, 29
amino acids, 33, 34, 54
amyotrophic lateral sclerosis, 17
anabolic, 25
androgen formation, 50
anemia, 20, 45, 51, 52
Antibody,22, 23
anticancer effects, 58
anti-cancer treatments, 55
anti-inflammatory, 33, 34, 35, 36, 37, 49, 50, 58
apoptosis, 49
arthritic, 10, 23, 43
arthritis, 8, 9, 11, 35, 36, 37, 38, 39, 40, 41, 63
atopic dermatitis, 25
atopy, 25
autoimmune diseases, 41, 49
blood cell production,, 6, 8, 18, 44
blood pressure, 47
bone marrow depression, 19
bones, 23, 31, 33, 34, 36, 41, 63
brain, 13, 14, 16, 56, 59
cancer, 54, 55, 56, 57, 58, 59, 62
carcinomas, 57
cardioprotection, 45, 46
Cardiovascular, 6, 8, 46, 63
cartilage, 31, 33, 34, 36, 37, 38, 41, 43, 47,59 60, 61
chemotherapy, 18, 57, 59
cholesterol, 47
chondroitin sulfate, 33, 37, 38
circulation, 46
collagen, 31,33, 37, 41, 42
Degenerative Myelopathy, 17
diabetes, 8, 16, 49, 56
DNA, 57
Dr. John Prudden, 59
EGF, 14, 51, 56, 57
EGFR, 56
Ehrlichia, 19
Ehrlichiosis, 19
Endurance, 47, 48
Essential fatty acids, 34
estrogen replacement therapies., 50
FGF, 15
fibroblasts, 41, 47

follicular receptor dysregulation, 27
fracture, 9, 10, 40, 47
fracture healing, 40, 47
glucosamine, 2, 33, 38, 39
glycosaminoglycans, 33, 37
Glycosphingolipids, 33
Growth factors, 14, 15, 16, 17, 34, 51, 57
healing wounds, 23, 24
hemoglobin, 22, 51
hip dysplasia, 36
Hodgkin's Disease, 59
Hyaluronic acid, 33
IGF-1, 16, 17, 54, 57
immune function, 22, 48, 58, 59
immune stimulant, 23
Immuno modulation, 8
immunomodulators, 22
incontinence, 50
joint, 6, 8, 11, 32, 33, 35, 36, 37, 41
joint pain, 11,32
kidney:, 11, 12, 32, 37, 48, 55, 58
liver, 11, 26, 32, 37, 47, 48, 59
Lou Gehrig's disease, 16
lymphoma, 49
mammary hyperplasia., 50
Marfan syndrome, 56
mending bones, 23
minerals, 34
monoamine-oxidase inhibitors, 34
multiple sclerosis, 16, 41, 56
muscle strength, 15
muscle tissue, 16, 63
muscular atrophy, 50
Mycoplasma hemofelis, 20
myelin sheaths, 16
myocardial infarction, 46
nerve function, 16
nerve regeneration, 17
nerve tissue, 15, 17, 18, 63
NGF, 15
oncogenesis, 56
osteoarthritis, 35, 36, 37, 38, 39, 41,
osteoarthrosis, 42, 43
oxidative stress, 49
pain., 9, 11, 12, 35, 36
Phosphorus, 34
Polysaccharides, 34, 46, 49, 50
Prostaglandins, 34, 50
psoriasis, 26
red blood cell, 6,8,18,44
regenerate nerve tissue, 17
rheumatoid arthritis, 41

ringworm, 28
seborrhea, 27
spinal-cord injuries, 62
stem cells, 13, 14, 61, 62
stress responses, 44
stroke, 46, 62
surgery, 6, 8, 35, 38, 40, 49, 59, 63
T cell, 13, 25, 49, 56
thymus, 6, 22, 41
tissue regeneration, 14, 50
tissue Repair, 46
Transforming Growth Factor, 14, 55, 56
trauma, 10, 13, 23, 36, 62, 63
tumor, 45, 54, 55, 56, 57
ulcerative colitis, 57
ulcers, 11, 2, 32
uveitis, 41, 49
VEGF, 15
vitiligo, 49
whiplash injuries, 18
white blood cells, 22, 32, 58
wound healing, 8, 23, 24, 44, 46, 47, 49, 51
wounds, 23, 24, 25, 51, 63

Endnotes

---

[1] www.vitaminsinamerica.com/news/velvet.htm

[2] Cheng H, Randolph A. et.al., "Characterization of Insulin-Like Growth Factor-1 and Its Receptor and Binding Proteins in Transected Nerves and Cultured Schwann Cells", Journal of Neurochemistry Lippioncoot-Raven Publishers, Philadelphia 1996 pp. 525-537 International Society for Neurochemistry,Univ of Michigan Dept of Neurology and Neuroscience Program Ann Arbor Michigan.

[3] Lu L, Wang K, et.al., "Effect of velvet antler polypeptide on peripheral nerve regeneration.", Zhongguo Xie Fu Chong Jian Wai Ke Za Zhi, 2008;22(12):1458-61, Chinese PubMed PMID: 19137890.

[4] Hansson H., Dahlin L., et.al., "Evidence indicating trophic importance of IGF-1 in regenerating peripheral nerves Acta Physiologica.", Scandinavica Volume 126, Issue 4, pages 609–614, April 1986.

[5] Takikawa K, Kokubu N, et.al., "Studies of experimental whiplash injury II. Evaluation of pantui extracts, Pantocrin as a remedy." Folia Pharmacol. Japan;68:473-488.

[6] Suttie, Haines, Li (2004), "Advances in Antler Science and Product Technology," 2nd International Symposium on Antler Science and Product Technology Deer Industry New Zealand.

[7] Gu, LiJuan. "Effects of Red Deer Antlers on Cutaneous Wound Healing in Full-thickness Rat Models." The Asian-Australasian Journal of Animal Sciences 21.2 (2008): 277-90. Web.

[8] Sunwoo, H.H; T. Nakano; RJ. Hudson; J.S. Sim. "Isolation, characterization and localization of glycosaminesin growing antlers of wapiti (Cervus elaphus)". Comparative Biochemistry and Physiology Part B 1998:273-283.

[9] Moreau M, Dupuis J, Bonneau NH, Lécuyer M, *Clinical evaluation of a powder of quality deer velvet antler for the treatment of osteoarthrosis in dogs*. Can Vet J. 2004 Feb;45(2):133-9.

[10] Zhang ZQ, Wang Y, Zhang H, et al., *Anti-inflammatory effects of pilose antler peptide.*, Zhongguo Yao Li Xue-Bao., 1994.

[11] Kang, W S., "Influence of antler (deer horn) on the mesenteric mast cells of rates exposed to heat, cold or electric shock." J. Cathol. Med. College 1970; 19:1-9.

[12] Yudin, A. M. and Y L. Dubryakov 1974. "A guide for the preparation and storage of uncalcified male antlers as a medicinal raw mate-

rial. In: Reindeer Antlers," Academy of Sciences of the USSR, Vladivostock: Far East Science Center.

[13] Church, J.S. *Velvet Antler: Its historical medical use, performance enhancing effects and pharmacology*. Elk Tech International Research Centre, http:/www.elktech.com/research.htm. 1999.

[14] Ibid.

[15] Suttie, J.M.; PF Fennessy; S.R. Haines; M. Sadighi; D.R. Kerr; C. lssacs. "The New Zealand velvet antler industry: Background and research findings." International symposium on Cervi Parvum Cornu. KSP Proceedings. 1994; 86-I 35.

[16] http:/www.elktech.com/research.htm. 1999.

[17] Sunwoo-HH; Sim-JS, "Potential uses of velvet antler as nutraceuticals, functional and medical foods in the West", Journal-of-Nutraceuticals,-Functional-and-Medical-Foods, 2000, 2: 3, 5-23; 38 ref.

[18] Sung-HG; Kim-DK; Shin-HT, "Influence of powdered velvet antler on growth and intestinal organ development in Sprague-Dawley Rats.", Journal-of-Animal-Science-and-Technology, 2003, 45: 5, 749-758; 33 ref.

[19] Chen J., Woodbury M, et.al.,"Dietary Supplementa-tion of Femail Rats with Elk Velvet Antler Improves Physical and Neurolocical Development of Offspring," Evidence-Based Complementary and Alternative Medicine Volume 2012, Article ID 640680 7 pages.

[20] Church, J.S., *Velvet Antler: Its historical medical use, performance enhancing effects and pharmacology*. Elk Tech International Research Centre. 1999.

[21] Shao M., Wang S. et.al.,"The effects of velvet antler of deer on cardiac functions of rats with heart failure following myocardial infarction," Evidence-Based Complementary and Alternative Medicine, vol.2012, Article ID 825056 5 pages 2012.

[22] Price J. and Allen S., "Exploring the mechanisms regulating regeneration of deer antlers," Philos Trans R Soc Lond B Biol Sci., 2004 May 29; 359(1445): 809–822.

[23] Seok-Seon Roh, Min-Ho Lee, M.S.,et.al., *Stimulation of the Extracellular Matrix Production in Dermal Fibroblasts by Velvet Antler Extract,* Ann Dermatol, Vol. 22, No. 2, 2010.

[24] Wang BX, Chen XG, Xu HB, Zhang W, Zhang J. *Effect of polyamines isolated from pilose antler (PASPA) on RNA polymerase activities in mouse liver.* Yao Hsueh Hsueh Pao . 1990;25:652-657. / Ha H,

---

Yoon SH, et al., "Study for new hapatotropic agent from natural resources. I. Effect of antler and old antler on liver injury induced by benzopyrene in rats," Nihon Eiyo Shokuryo Gakkai Shi., Food & Nutrition 1990;23:9.

[25] Zhou QL, Guo YJ, Wang LJ, Wang Y, Liu YQ, Wang Y, Wang BX., *Velvet antler polypeptides promoted proliferation of chondrocytes and osteoblast precursors and fracture healing*. Research Centre of New Drug, Changchun College of Traditional Chinese Medicine, China. / Faucheux-C; Nesbitt-SA; Horton-MA; Price-JS, "Cells in regenerating deer antler cartilage provide a microenvironment that supports osteoclast differentiation,"Journal-of-Experimental-Biology. 2001, 204: 3, 443-455.

[26] Broeder, C.E.; Percival, R.; Quindry, J.; Panton, L.; Wills, T.; Browder, K.D.; Earnest, C.; Almada, A.; Haines, S. R.; Suttie, J.M., "The effects of New Zealand deer velvet antler supplementation on body composition, strength, and maximal aerobic and anaerobic performance." In: Suttie, J.M.; Haines, S.R.; Li C. (eds.), "Advances in Antler Science and Product Technology", Taieri Print, Fairfield, Dunedin, New Zealand. 2004 pp 161-165. / Gerrard, D.F., G.G. Sleivert, A.Goulding, S.R. Haines, and J.N. Suttie. Clinical Evaluation of New Zealand Deer Velvet Antler on Muscle Strength and Endurance and Healthy Male University Athletes, Burgio P, *The Velvet antler: Its Medicinal application, factors affecting growth, and biochemical analysis North American Elk*(1997) 8 (4) p.76.

[27] Wang, B.X.; X.G. Chen; W Zhang., *Influence of the active compounds isolated from pilose antler on syntheses of protein and RNA in mouse liver.*, [Article in Chinese] Yao Hsueh Hsueh Pao 1990;25(5):321-325.

[28] Kuo C., Wang T, et.al., "Effect of the Velvet Antler of Formosan Sambar Deer (Cervus unicolor swinhoei) on the Prevention of an Allergic Airway Response in Mice.", Evidence-Based Complementary and Alternative Medicine Volume 2013 Article ID 481318 10 pages.

[29] Ablamunits V., Petrov V. "Costimulatory Effect of Velvet Antler on Proliferation of Human T Lymphocytes Popular Asian treatment may modulate immune response to antigens" Natural Medicine Journal March 2012 Vol. 4 Issue 3.
http://naturalmedicinejournal.com/journal/2012-03/costimulatory-effect-velvet-antler-proliferation-human-t-lymphocytes/

[30] Cooney A., *A Review of Scientific Literature on the Health Benefits of Velvet Antler* (2001) 34-37

---

[31] Kamen B, "The remarkable healing power of velvet antler." Nutrition Encounter Novata, CA 1999 pg 152

[32] Wang BX, Liu AJ, Cheng XJ, Wang QG, Wei GR, Cui JC., *Anti-ulcer action of the polysaccharides isolated from pilose antler*. Yao Hsueh Hsueh Pao , 1985;20:321-325.

[33] Church, J.S., *Velvet Antler: Its historical medical use, performance enhancing effects and pharmacology*. Elk Tech International Research Centre, http:/www.elktech.com/research.htm. 1999.

[34] Mikler JR, Theoret CL, High JC., "Wound Healing Effects of topical elk velvet antler on cutaneous wound healing in streptozotocin-induced diabetic rats." [Canada: Department of Pharmacology, College of Medicine, University of Saskatchewan, Saskatoon, Saskatchewan, Canada.]

[35] Kim KL, Shin MK, Lee HI, Kim WH and Lee, "St Deer Velvet Benefit - Tested For Treatment of Anemia. Effect of several kinds of antler (Cervi cornu) on the erythro-cytic activity in experimentally induced anaemic rabbits." Samwon Commercial Company, Korea Trading Agents Associations, Seoul. Undated.

[36] D. Zur B.SC/B.V.SC, A.Reason DVM, A. Kafri DVM

[37]Wang, B., "Advances in research of chemistry, pharmacology and clinical application of pilose antler." Proceedings of the 1996 International Symposium on Deer Science and Deer Products. 1996; I4-31. / Church, J.S., "Velvet Antler: Its historical medical use, performance enhancing effects and pharmacology." Elk Tech International Research Centre, http:/www.elktech.com/research.htm. 1999.

[38] Editor, North American Elk Research links velvet antler to multi-billion dollar dietary supplement industry. North American Elk 1998 Fall:121-123

[39] Fennessy P 1991, *Velvet antler: the produce and pharma-cology. Proc.Deer Course for Veterinarians* (Deer Branch of the NZ Vet Assoc), 8 pp.169-80.

[40] Kim DH, Han SB, Yu KU, et al., *Antitumor activity of fermented antler on sarcoma 180 in mice*., Yakhak Hoeji. 1994. / Church, J.S., *Velvet Antler: Its historical medical use, performance enhancing effects and pharmacology*., Elk Tech International Research Centre. 1999.

[41] Editor, North American Elk, "Research links velvet antler to multi-billion dollar dietary supplement industry." North American Elk 1998 Fall:121-123

---

[42] Suttie, J et.al.,"Reduction in Side-Effects of Anti-Cancer Treatments." New Zealand Velvet Research, Sep1997

[43] Suttie, JM., et al. "The Velvet Antler Industry: Background and Research Findings. International Symposium on Cervi Parvum Cornu." Abdo, J., ed. The Korean Society of Pharmacology, Seoul, Korea. Oct. 7, 1994.

[44] Wang B., "Advances in Research of Chemistry, Pharmacology and Clinical Application of Pilose Antler." Proceedings of the 1996 International Symposium on Deer Science and Deer Products, I4-31.Extracts of deer antler have reduced tumor cell growth./ Yudin A, et al., "A Guide for the Preparation and Storage of Uncalcified Male Antlers as a Medicinal Raw Material." In: Reindeer Antlers, Academy of Sciences of the USSR. Vladivostock: Far East Science Center; 1974.

[45] Sim JS, et al., "Canadian scientists study velvet antler for arthritis treatment." Can Elk Deer Farmer, Winter 1999:39-40./ Goss RJ, "Future directions in antler research," Anat Rec. 1995;241:291-302.

[46] Prudden John F.; "The Treatment of Human Cancer with Agents Prepared From Bovine Cartilage," Journal of Biological Response Modifiers4 (6): 551-84(1985).

[47] Bowen, Tim. "Deer Antlers Hold Clues To Stem Cell Research." *Medical News Today*. MediLexicon, Intl., 15 Jan. 2006. Web. 20 Mar. 2015 http://www.medicalnewstoday.com/releases/36174.php

[48] "Multipotent stem cells in deer antler may have regenerative uses in veterinary medicine," Cell Transplantation Center of Excellence for Aging and Brain Repair, http://www.news-medical.net/news/20130320/Multipotent-stem-cells-in-deer-antler-may-have-regenerative-uses-in-veterinary-medicine.aspx Published on March 20, 2013

Other Books by Safe Goods

Super Nutrition for Dogs n' Cats

Cancer Disarmed

Prevent Cancer, Strokes, Heart Attacks
and other Deadly Killers

Overcoming Senior Moments

Lower Blood Pressure without Drugs

Lower Cholesterol without Drugs

Effective Secret Solutions for Anxiety and Stress Relief

The Secrets of Staying Young

The ADD and ADHD Diet!

ADD, The Natural Approach

Testosterone is your Friend

The Natural Diabetes Cure

Velvet Antler

Eye Care Naturally

Rx for Computer Eyes

Feeling Younger with Homeopathic HGH